Summer Day Essential Oils
37 Legendary Diffuser Blends To Bring The Summer Mood Into Your Home

Table of content

4

Introduction

Summer is here and you are more than ready. It seemed the winter would never end, and now that the sunshine is out, you are ready to celebrate. Whether you are going to the beach, having fun with friends and family, or you are simply living it up flying solo, you know this is your favorite time of year.

What better way to enjoy the summer than to enrich your home with the best scents you can imagine? You know you love the fresh air, and you want to celebrate that with a richness in your home like you haven't had in months.

And where are you going to get this richness? Through essential oils, of course.

You know you love the blends, and you know you want nothing but the most natural options for you and your family.

And to get those blends, you have come to the right place. Let me show you everything you need to know to have the best blends for your home diffuser, and fill your house with scents so rich, you will feel like you live in paradise.

Let's get started.

Chapter 1 – The Blends

Make each of the blends as they are, or experiment with the different scents to find your own!

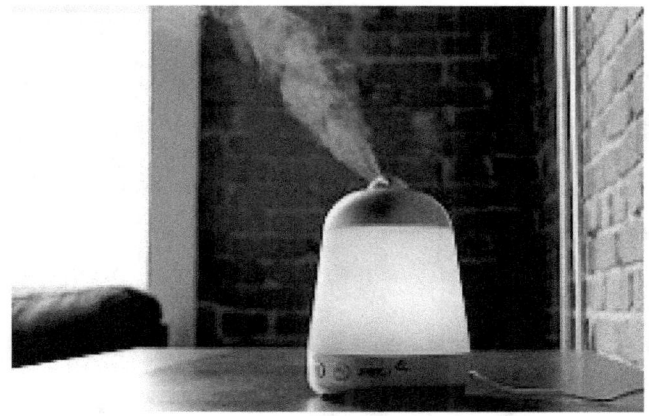

Summer Sunset
What you will need:

8 drops lavender

8 drops rose

8 drops lemon

Directions:

Mix the blend immediately before you place in your diffuser. Make sure you fill your diffuser according to the instructions on the packaging – don't overfill and don't add too much oil, many diffusers only require a few drops of oil mixed with water to work properly, so make sure you know what your particular diffuser needs.

Plug in and turn on your diffuser, and breathe in the rich sent of your chosen blend. Again, follow the directions on your diffuser, and run for the allotted amount of time on the packaging.

Can be used as often as you like. Try multiple diffusers for a rich scent throughout your entire home!

The Cricket Blend

What you will need:

8 drops wheatgrass

7 drops persimmon

3 drops lavender

Directions:

Mix the blend immediately before you place in your diffuser. Make sure you fill your diffuser according to the instructions on the packaging – don't overfill and don't add too much oil, many diffusers only require a few drops of oil mixed with water to work properly, so make sure you know what your particular diffuser needs.

Plug in and turn on your diffuser, and breathe in the rich sent of your chosen blend. Again, follow the directions on your diffuser, and run for the allotted amount of time on the packaging.

Can be used as often as you like. Try multiple diffusers for a rich scent throughout your entire home!

Early Mornings

What you will need:

11 drops lemon

10 drops grapefruit

10 drops ylang ylang

Directions:

Mix the blend immediately before you place in your diffuser. Make sure you fill your diffuser according to the instructions on the packaging – don't overfill and don't add too much oil, many diffusers only require a few drops of oil mixed with water to work properly, so make sure you know what your particular diffuser needs.

Plug in and turn on your diffuser, and breathe in the rich sent of your chosen blend. Again, follow the directions on your diffuser, and run for the allotted amount of time on the packaging.

Can be used as often as you like. Try multiple diffusers for a rich scent throughout your entire home!

The Crack of Dawn

What you will need:

10 drops cacao

10 drops vanilla

10 drops cardamom

Directions:

Mix the blend immediately before you place in your diffuser. Make sure you fill your diffuser according to the instructions on the packaging – don't overfill and don't add too much oil, many diffusers only require a few drops of oil mixed with water to work properly, so make sure you know what your particular diffuser needs.

Plug in and turn on your diffuser, and breathe in the rich sent of your chosen blend. Again, follow the directions on your diffuser, and run for the allotted amount of time on the packaging.

Can be used as often as you like. Try multiple diffusers for a rich scent throughout your entire home!

Meditation

What you will need:

10 drops myrrh

10 drops frankincense

10 drops rose

Directions:

Mix the blend immediately before you place in your diffuser. Make sure you fill your diffuser according to the instructions on the packaging – don't overfill and don't add too much oil, many diffusers only require a few drops of oil mixed with water to work properly, so make sure you know what your particular diffuser needs.

Plug in and turn on your diffuser, and breathe in the rich sent of your chosen blend. Again, follow the directions on your diffuser, and run for the allotted amount of time on the packaging.

Can be used as often as you like. Try multiple diffusers for a rich scent throughout your entire home!

The Chickadee's Song
What you will need:

10 drops pine

10 drops cedar

12 drops sandalwood

Directions:

Mix the blend immediately before you place in your diffuser. Make sure you fill your diffuser according to the instructions on the packaging – don't overfill and

don't add too much oil, many diffusers only require a few drops of oil mixed with water to work properly, so make sure you know what your particular diffuser needs.

Plug in and turn on your diffuser, and breathe in the rich sent of your chosen blend. Again, follow the directions on your diffuser, and run for the allotted amount of time on the packaging.

Can be used as often as you like. Try multiple diffusers for a rich scent throughout your entire home!

Summertime Gladness

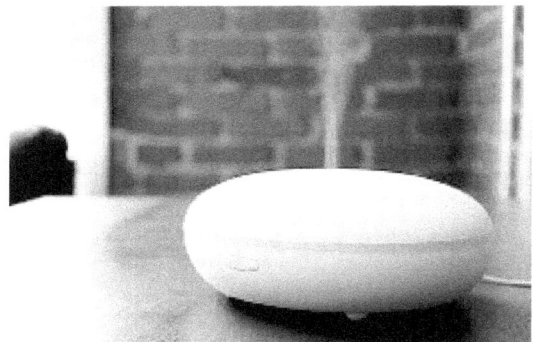

What you will need:

10 drops rosewood

10 drops basil

8 drops chamomile

Directions:

Mix the blend immediately before you place in your diffuser. Make sure you fill your diffuser according to the instructions on the packaging – don't overfill and don't add too much oil, many diffusers only require a few drops of oil mixed with water to work properly, so make sure you know what your particular diffuser needs.

Plug in and turn on your diffuser, and breathe in the rich sent of your chosen blend. Again, follow the directions on your diffuser, and run for the allotted amount of time on the packaging.

Can be used as often as you like. Try multiple diffusers for a rich scent throughout your entire home!

Splash
What you will need:

10 drops myrrh

8 drops bergamot

8 drops cinnamon

Directions:

Mix the blend immediately before you place in your diffuser. Make sure you fill your diffuser according to the instructions on the packaging – don't overfill and don't add too much oil, many diffusers only require a few drops of oil mixed with water to work properly, so make sure you know what your particular diffuser needs.

Plug in and turn on your diffuser, and breathe in the rich sent of your chosen blend. Again, follow the directions on your diffuser, and run for the allotted amount of time on the packaging.

Can be used as often as you like. Try multiple diffusers for a rich scent throughout your entire home!

Midsummer Night's Dream

What you will need:

8 drops sunflower

8 drops cedar

8 drops neem

Directions:

Mix the blend immediately before you place in your diffuser. Make sure you fill your diffuser according to the instructions on the packaging – don't overfill and

don't add too much oil, many diffusers only require a few drops of oil mixed with water to work properly, so make sure you know what your particular diffuser needs.

Plug in and turn on your diffuser, and breathe in the rich sent of your chosen blend. Again, follow the directions on your diffuser, and run for the allotted amount of time on the packaging.

Can be used as often as you like. Try multiple diffusers for a rich scent throughout your entire home!

Kiss of the Breeze

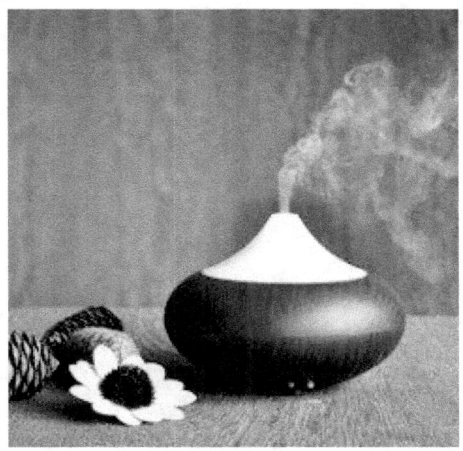

What you will need:

10 drops orange

10 drops lemon

12 drops grapefruit

Directions:

Mix the blend immediately before you place in your diffuser. Make sure you fill your diffuser according to the instructions on the packaging – don't overfill and don't add too much oil, many diffusers only require a few drops of oil mixed with water to work properly, so make sure you know what your particular diffuser needs.

Plug in and turn on your diffuser, and breathe in the rich sent of your chosen blend. Again, follow the directions on your diffuser, and run for the allotted amount of time on the packaging.

Can be used as often as you like. Try multiple diffusers for a rich scent throughout your entire home!

Warmth
What you will need:

10 drops pine

10 drops orange

8 drops cinnamon

Directions:

Mix the blend immediately before you place in your diffuser. Make sure you fill your diffuser according to the instructions on the packaging – don't overfill and don't add too much oil, many diffusers only require a few drops of oil mixed with water to work properly, so make sure you know what your particular diffuser needs.

Plug in and turn on your diffuser, and breathe in the rich sent of your chosen blend. Again, follow the directions on your diffuser, and run for the allotted amount of time on the packaging.

Can be used as often as you like. Try multiple diffusers for a rich scent throughout your entire home!

Friends and Family

What you will need:

10 drops rose

8 drops juniper berry

8 drops jasmine

Directions:

Mix the blend immediately before you place in your diffuser. Make sure you fill your diffuser according to the instructions on the packaging – don't overfill and don't add too much oil, many diffusers only require a few drops of oil mixed with water to work properly, so make sure you know what your particular diffuser needs.

Plug in and turn on your diffuser, and breathe in the rich sent of your chosen blend. Again, follow the directions on your diffuser, and run for the allotted amount of time on the packaging.

Can be used as often as you like. Try multiple diffusers for a rich scent throughout your entire home!

Fresh Air

What you will need:

10 drops myrrh

8 drops sandalwood

8 drops geranium

Directions:

Mix the blend immediately before you place in your diffuser. Make sure you fill your diffuser according to the instructions on the packaging – don't overfill and don't add too much oil, many diffusers only require a few drops of oil mixed with water to work properly, so make sure you know what your particular diffuser needs.

Plug in and turn on your diffuser, and breathe in the rich sent of your chosen blend. Again, follow the directions on your diffuser, and run for the allotted amount of time on the packaging.

Can be used as often as you like. Try multiple diffusers for a rich scent throughout your entire home!

Top of the Morning

What you will need:

18

10 drops lemon

10 drops lemongrass

10 drops grapefruit

Directions:

Mix the blend immediately before you place in your diffuser. Make sure you fill your diffuser according to the instructions on the packaging – don't overfill and

don't add too much oil, many diffusers only require a few drops of oil mixed with water to work properly, so make sure you know what your particular diffuser needs.

Plug in and turn on your diffuser, and breathe in the rich sent of your chosen blend. Again, follow the directions on your diffuser, and run for the allotted amount of time on the packaging.

Can be used as often as you like. Try multiple diffusers for a rich scent throughout your entire home!

Sunshine and Smoothies
What you will need:

8 drops eucalyptus

8 drops spearmint

9 drops peppermint

Directions:

Mix the blend immediately before you place in your diffuser. Make sure you fill your diffuser according to the instructions on the packaging – don't overfill and don't add too much oil, many diffusers only require a few drops of oil mixed with water to work properly, so make sure you know what your particular diffuser needs.

Plug in and turn on your diffuser, and breathe in the rich sent of your chosen blend. Again, follow the directions on your diffuser, and run for the allotted amount of time on the packaging.

Can be used as often as you like. Try multiple diffusers for a rich scent throughout your entire home!

Girlfriend Blend

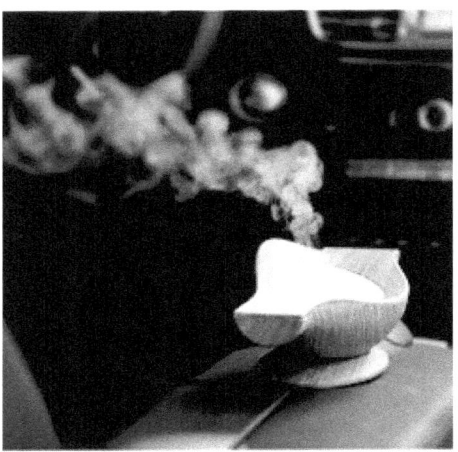

What you will need:

12 drops lavender

8 drops sage

8 drops clary sage

Directions:

Mix the blend immediately before you place in your diffuser. Make sure you fill your diffuser according to the instructions on the packaging – don't overfill and don't add too much oil, many diffusers only require a few drops of oil mixed with water to work properly, so make sure you know what your particular diffuser needs.

Plug in and turn on your diffuser, and breathe in the rich sent of your chosen blend. Again, follow the directions on your diffuser, and run for the allotted amount of time on the packaging.

Can be used as often as you like. Try multiple diffusers for a rich scent throughout your entire home!

In My Garden
What you will need:

10 drops orange

8 drops spearmint

7 drops ylang ylang

Directions:

Mix the blend immediately before you place in your diffuser. Make sure you fill your diffuser according to the instructions on the packaging – don't overfill and don't add too much oil, many diffusers only require a few drops of oil mixed with water to work properly, so make sure you know what your particular diffuser needs.

Plug in and turn on your diffuser, and breathe in the rich sent of your chosen blend. Again, follow the directions on your diffuser, and run for the allotted amount of time on the packaging.

Can be used as often as you like. Try multiple diffusers for a rich scent throughout your entire home!

The Bee's Knees
What you will need:

10 drops jasmine

9 drops vanilla

8 drops cinnamon

Directions:

Mix the blend immediately before you place in your diffuser. Make sure you fill your diffuser according to the instructions on the packaging – don't overfill and don't add too much oil, many diffusers only require a few drops of oil mixed with water to work properly, so make sure you know what your particular diffuser needs.

Plug in and turn on your diffuser, and breathe in the rich sent of your chosen blend. Again, follow the directions on your diffuser, and run for the allotted amount of time on the packaging.

Can be used as often as you like. Try multiple diffusers for a rich scent throughout your entire home!

Green Fields
What you will need:

10 drops neem

11 drops wheatgrass

8 drops lime

Directions:

Mix the blend immediately before you place in your diffuser. Make sure you fill your diffuser according to the instructions on the packaging – don't overfill and

don't add too much oil, many diffusers only require a few drops of oil mixed with water to work properly, so make sure you know what your particular diffuser needs.

Plug in and turn on your diffuser, and breathe in the rich sent of your chosen blend. Again, follow the directions on your diffuser, and run for the allotted amount of time on the packaging.

Can be used as often as you like. Try multiple diffusers for a rich scent throughout your entire home!

Happiness

What you will need:

10 drops grapefruit

8 drops peppermint

8 drops eucalyptus

Directions:

Mix the blend immediately before you place in your diffuser. Make sure you fill your diffuser according to the instructions on the packaging – don't overfill and don't add too much oil, many diffusers only require a few drops of oil mixed with water to work properly, so make sure you know what your particular diffuser needs.

Plug in and turn on your diffuser, and breathe in the rich sent of your chosen blend. Again, follow the directions on your diffuser, and run for the allotted amount of time on the packaging.

Can be used as often as you like. Try multiple diffusers for a rich scent throughout your entire home!

Thunderstorm

What you will need:

10 drops pine

10 drops wintergreen

8 drops sandalwood

Directions:

Mix the blend immediately before you place in your diffuser. Make sure you fill your diffuser according to the instructions on the packaging – don't overfill and don't add too much oil, many diffusers only require a few drops of oil mixed with water to work properly, so make sure you know what your particular diffuser needs.

Plug in and turn on your diffuser, and breathe in the rich sent of your chosen blend. Again, follow the directions on your diffuser, and run for the allotted amount of time on the packaging.

Can be used as often as you like. Try multiple diffusers for a rich scent throughout your entire home!

Lemonade Stand
What you will need:

12 drops lemon

8 drops lime

5 drops orange

Directions:

Mix the blend immediately before you place in your diffuser. Make sure you fill your diffuser according to the instructions on the packaging – don't overfill and don't add too much oil, many diffusers only require a few drops of oil mixed with water to work properly, so make sure you know what your particular diffuser needs.

Plug in and turn on your diffuser, and breathe in the rich sent of your chosen blend. Again, follow the directions on your diffuser, and run for the allotted amount of time on the packaging.

Can be used as often as you like. Try multiple diffusers for a rich scent throughout your entire home!

Kiss of the Night

What you will need:

12 drops rose

8 drops cedar

9 drops cinnamon

Directions:

Mix the blend immediately before you place in your diffuser. Make sure you fill your diffuser according to the instructions on the packaging – don't overfill and don't add too much oil, many diffusers only require a few drops of oil mixed with water to work properly, so make sure you know what your particular diffuser needs.

Plug in and turn on your diffuser, and breathe in the rich sent of your chosen blend. Again, follow the directions on your diffuser, and run for the allotted amount of time on the packaging.

Can be used as often as you like. Try multiple diffusers for a rich scent throughout your entire home!

Play Date

What you will need:

10 drops cinnamon

10 drops basil

8 drops tea tree

Directions:

Mix the blend immediately before you place in your diffuser. Make sure you fill your diffuser according to the instructions on the packaging – don't overfill and don't add too much oil, many diffusers only require a few drops of oil mixed with water to work properly, so make sure you know what your particular diffuser needs.

Plug in and turn on your diffuser, and breathe in the rich sent of your chosen blend. Again, follow the directions on your diffuser, and run for the allotted amount of time on the packaging.

Can be used as often as you like. Try multiple diffusers for a rich scent throughout your entire home!

Picnic in the Park

What you will need:

11 drops lemon

10 drops oregano

10 drops grapefruit

Directions:

Mix the blend immediately before you place in your diffuser. Make sure you fill your diffuser according to the instructions on the packaging – don't overfill and don't add too much oil, many diffusers only require a few drops of oil mixed with water to work properly, so make sure you know what your particular diffuser needs.

Plug in and turn on your diffuser, and breathe in the rich sent of your chosen blend. Again, follow the directions on your diffuser, and run for the allotted amount of time on the packaging.

Can be used as often as you like. Try multiple diffusers for a rich scent throughout your entire home!

Blue Skies

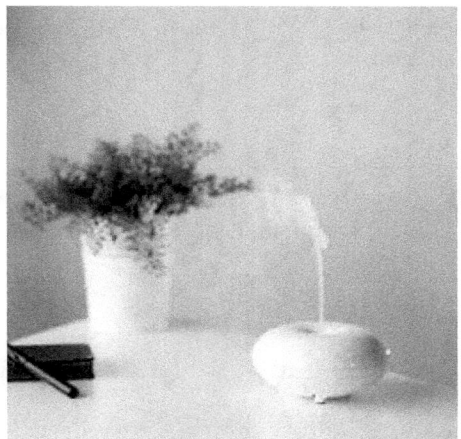

What you will need:

10 drops cedar

8 drops frankincense

2 drops tea tree

Directions:

Mix the blend immediately before you place in your diffuser. Make sure you fill your diffuser according to the instructions on the packaging – don't overfill and

don't add too much oil, many diffusers only require a few drops of oil mixed with water to work properly, so make sure you know what your particular diffuser needs.

Plug in and turn on your diffuser, and breathe in the rich sent of your chosen blend. Again, follow the directions on your diffuser, and run for the allotted amount of time on the packaging.

Can be used as often as you like. Try multiple diffusers for a rich scent throughout your entire home!

School's Out

What you will need:

9 drops jasmine

8 drops myrrh

8 drops chamomile

Directions:

Mix the blend immediately before you place in your diffuser. Make sure you fill your diffuser according to the instructions on the packaging – don't overfill and don't add too much oil, many diffusers only require a few drops of oil mixed with water to work properly, so make sure you know what your particular diffuser needs.

Plug in and turn on your diffuser, and breathe in the rich sent of your chosen blend. Again, follow the directions on your diffuser, and run for the allotted amount of time on the packaging.

Can be used as often as you like. Try multiple diffusers for a rich scent throughout your entire home!

Misty Mountain

What you will need:

8 drops eucalyptus

7 drops wintergreen

8 drops spearmint

Directions:

Mix the blend immediately before you place in your diffuser. Make sure you fill your diffuser according to the instructions on the packaging – don't overfill and don't add too much oil, many diffusers only require a few drops of oil mixed with water to work properly, so make sure you know what your particular diffuser needs.

Plug in and turn on your diffuser, and breathe in the rich sent of your chosen blend. Again, follow the directions on your diffuser, and run for the allotted amount of time on the packaging.

Can be used as often as you like. Try multiple diffusers for a rich scent throughout your entire home!

Rainy Days

What you will need:

12 drops bergamot

8 drops basil

4 drops pine

Directions:

Mix the blend immediately before you place in your diffuser. Make sure you fill your diffuser according to the instructions on the packaging – don't overfill and don't add too much oil, many diffusers only require a few drops of oil mixed with water to work properly, so make sure you know what your particular diffuser needs.

Plug in and turn on your diffuser, and breathe in the rich sent of your chosen blend. Again, follow the directions on your diffuser, and run for the allotted amount of time on the packaging.

Can be used as often as you like. Try multiple diffusers for a rich scent throughout your entire home!

Summer Vacation
What you will need:

10 drops neem

10 drops vetiver

3 drops goldenseal

Directions:

Mix the blend immediately before you place in your diffuser. Make sure you fill your diffuser according to the instructions on the packaging – don't overfill and don't add too much oil, many diffusers only require a few drops of oil mixed with water to work properly, so make sure you know what your particular diffuser needs.

Plug in and turn on your diffuser, and breathe in the rich sent of your chosen blend. Again, follow the directions on your diffuser, and run for the allotted amount of time on the packaging.

Can be used as often as you like. Try multiple diffusers for a rich scent throughout your entire home!

It's an Herb
What you will need:

12 drops basil

10 drops parsley

8 drops oregano

Directions:

Mix the blend immediately before you place in your diffuser. Make sure you fill your diffuser according to the instructions on the packaging – don't overfill and don't add too much oil, many diffusers only require a few drops of oil mixed with water to work properly, so make sure you know what your particular diffuser needs.

Plug in and turn on your diffuser, and breathe in the rich sent of your chosen blend. Again, follow the directions on your diffuser, and run for the allotted amount of time on the packaging.

Can be used as often as you like. Try multiple diffusers for a rich scent throughout your entire home!

Ocean Fun

What you will need:

12 drops sandalwood

8 drops helichrysum

2 drops tea tree

Directions:

Mix the blend immediately before you place in your diffuser. Make sure you fill your diffuser according to the instructions on the packaging – don't overfill and don't add too much oil, many diffusers only require a few drops of oil mixed with water to work properly, so make sure you know what your particular diffuser needs.

Plug in and turn on your diffuser, and breathe in the rich sent of your chosen blend. Again, follow the directions on your diffuser, and run for the allotted amount of time on the packaging.

Can be used as often as you like. Try multiple diffusers for a rich scent throughout your entire home!

Selfie

What you will need:

7 drops ylang ylang

5 drops jojoba

5 drops rose

Directions:

Mix the blend immediately before you place in your diffuser. Make sure you fill your diffuser according to the instructions on the packaging – don't overfill and don't add too much oil, many diffusers only require a few drops of oil mixed with water to work properly, so make sure you know what your particular diffuser needs.

Plug in and turn on your diffuser, and breathe in the rich sent of your chosen blend. Again, follow the directions on your diffuser, and run for the allotted amount of time on the packaging.

Can be used as often as you like. Try multiple diffusers for a rich scent throughout your entire home!

The Merry-Go-Round Blend

What you will need:

8 drops star anise

8 drops myrrh

7 drops geranium

Directions:

Mix the blend immediately before you place in your diffuser. Make sure you fill your diffuser according to the instructions on the packaging – don't overfill and don't add too much oil, many diffusers only require a few drops of oil mixed with water to work properly, so make sure you know what your particular diffuser needs.

Plug in and turn on your diffuser, and breathe in the rich sent of your chosen blend. Again, follow the directions on your diffuser, and run for the allotted amount of time on the packaging.

Can be used as often as you like. Try multiple diffusers for a rich scent throughout your entire home!

Trips and Treats
What you will need:

8 drops vetiver

8 drops juniper

8 drops jasmine

Directions:

Mix the blend immediately before you place in your diffuser. Make sure you fill your diffuser according to the instructions on the packaging – don't overfill and

don't add too much oil, many diffusers only require a few drops of oil mixed with water to work properly, so make sure you know what your particular diffuser needs.

Plug in and turn on your diffuser, and breathe in the rich sent of your chosen blend. Again, follow the directions on your diffuser, and run for the allotted amount of time on the packaging.

Can be used as often as you like. Try multiple diffusers for a rich scent throughout your entire home!

The Teeter Totter
What you will need:

10 drops chamomile

9 drops roman chamomile

8 drops geranium

Directions:

Mix the blend immediately before you place in your diffuser. Make sure you fill your diffuser according to the instructions on the packaging – don't overfill and

don't add too much oil, many diffusers only require a few drops of oil mixed with water to work properly, so make sure you know what your particular diffuser needs.

Plug in and turn on your diffuser, and breathe in the rich sent of your chosen blend. Again, follow the directions on your diffuser, and run for the allotted amount of time on the packaging.

Can be used as often as you like. Try multiple diffusers for a rich scent throughout your entire home!

Making Music

What you will need:

12 drops cardamom

8 drops juniper

8 drops peppermint

Directions:

Mix the blend immediately before you place in your diffuser. Make sure you fill your diffuser according to the instructions on the packaging – don't overfill and

don't add too much oil, many diffusers only require a few drops of oil mixed with water to work properly, so make sure you know what your particular diffuser needs.

Plug in and turn on your diffuser, and breathe in the rich sent of your chosen blend. Again, follow the directions on your diffuser, and run for the allotted amount of time on the packaging.

Can be used as often as you like. Try multiple diffusers for a rich scent throughout your entire home!

Conclusion

There you have it – a collection of summer blends that you can use in your home to bring in the warmth of the air. I hope this book inspires you to make the most of summer, and that you take the blends that you find here and showcase them in every room of your house.

You know you love this time of year, and with these glorious scents, you have everything you need to make sure that this summer is the freshest summer yet. Now get out there and catch some rays!

Have a happy summer – you deserve the best.

FREE Bonus Reminder

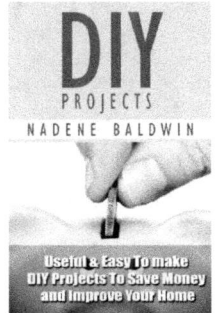

If you have not grabbed it yet, please go ahead and download your special bonus report *"DIY Projects. 13 Useful & Easy To Make DIY Projects To Save Money & Improve Your Home!"*

Simply Click the Button Below

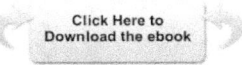

OR **Go to This Page**

http://diyhomecraft.com/free

BONUS #2: More Free & Discounted Books or Products

Do you want to receive more Free/Discounted Books or Products?

We have a mailing list where we send out our new Books or Products when they go free or with a discount on Amazon. Click on the link below to sign up for Free & Discount Book & Product Promotions.

=> Sign Up for Free & Discount Book & Product Promotions <=

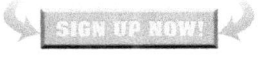

OR Go to this URL

http://zbit.ly/1WBb1Ek